GET FIT: A COMPREHENSIVE GUIDE TO A HEALTHIER LIFESTYLE

BY SIBUSISO NSIBANDE

Dedicated to all those who have decided to take control of their health and fitness, and to make positive changes in their lives. May this book inspire and guide you on your journey to a healthier and happier you.

Table of Contents

Introduction

Leading a healthy lifestyle is vital for maintaining optimal physical, mental, and emotional health. Exercise and proper nutrition are the two most critical components of a healthy lifestyle. They work together to keep your body in peak condition and help you feel your best.

Regular exercise has numerous benefits for your overall wellbeing. It can lower your risk of chronic diseases such as heart disease, stroke, and diabetes, which are leading causes of death worldwide. Additionally, exercise can help improve your mood, reduce stress, and boost your energy levels. Regular physical activity can also help you maintain a healthy weight, which is essential for preventing a variety of health problems.

Eating a balanced diet is equally important for maintaining good health. Consuming nutrient-dense foods, such as fruits, vegetables, whole grains, lean protein, and healthy fats, provides your body with the nutrients it needs to function at its best. Eating a healthy diet can help prevent chronic diseases, improve brain function, and boost your mood.

Unfortunately, many people struggle to incorporate exercise and healthy eating habits into their daily routine. Busy schedules, lack of motivation, and unhealthy habits can make it challenging to make lifestyle changes. That's why having a comprehensive guide to getting fit can be incredibly helpful.

In this book, we provide you with a step-by-step guide to help you achieve your fitness goals. We'll start by discussing the importance of setting goals, which can help keep you motivated and on track.

We'll also provide guidance on how to assess your current fitness level, so you can determine the best workout plan for your body.

Creating a workout plan that includes both aerobic and strength-training exercises is crucial for achieving your fitness goals. Aerobic exercises, such as running or cycling, can help improve your cardiovascular health, while strength training exercises, such as weightlifting, can help build muscle and improve bone density. It's also important to incorporate stretching and flexibility exercises into your routine to help prevent injury and improve mobility.

Making exercise a habit can be challenging, but it's essential for achieving your fitness goals. We'll provide you with tips on how to make exercise a part of your daily routine and keep yourself motivated. We'll also discuss the benefits of finding a workout partner or hiring a personal trainer to help keep you accountable and on track.

In addition to exercise, healthy eating habits are crucial for achieving optimal health. We'll discuss the importance of consuming nutrient-dense foods and limiting processed foods, added sugars, and saturated fats. We'll also provide tips on how to meal plan and prepare healthy meals, even when you're short on time.

Finally, we'll discuss the importance of tracking your progress and setting mini-goals to help keep you motivated. We'll also provide tips on how to avoid hitting a plateau and how to mix up your workouts to prevent boredom.

In conclusion, leading a healthy lifestyle is essential for achieving optimal health and wellbeing. Exercise and a balanced diet are the two most important components of a healthy lifestyle, and this book provides you with a comprehensive guide on how to incorporate both into your daily routine. Our aim is to give you the knowledge and tools you need to take control of your health and fitness and achieve your fitness goals. Remember, getting fit takes time, effort, and dedication, but the rewards are well worth it

Chapter 1:

The important of leading a healthy lifestyle

Maintaining a healthy lifestyle is crucial for our physical and mental well-being. A healthy lifestyle is characterized by a combination of regular exercise, a balanced diet, and adequate rest. This chapter aims to highlight the importance of leading a healthy lifestyle and the benefits of exercise and a balanced diet.

Firstly, leading a healthy lifestyle can prevent chronic diseases such as heart disease, diabetes, and stroke. It can also improve mental health and reduce the risk of depression and anxiety. Moreover, regular exercise and a balanced diet can improve sleep quality, energy levels, and self-esteem.

Secondly, regular exercise can improve cardiovascular health, muscular strength, flexibility, and body composition. Additionally, a balanced diet can provide the necessary nutrients to maintain and repair body tissues, support optimal brain function, and maintain a healthy weight.

Lastly, this book will provide a comprehensive guide on how to get fit, incorporating exercise and a balanced diet into your daily routine. This book aims to educate and empower individuals to take control of their health and fitness. The following chapters will cover topics such as setting goals, assessing fitness levels, creating a workout plan, making healthy lifestyle choices, and overcoming obstacles.

Importance of leading a healthy lifestyle

Maintaining a healthy lifestyle is critical for individuals of all ages, races, and genders. It involves making conscious and consistent efforts towards physical, mental, and emotional well-being. Living a healthy lifestyle has a wide range of benefits, some of which are discussed below.

1. Improved Physical Health

A healthy lifestyle can significantly improve physical health. Regular exercise and a balanced diet can help maintain a healthy weight, build strength and endurance, improve cardiovascular health, and prevent chronic diseases. Exercise helps improve bone density, reducing the risk of fractures and osteoporosis, while a balanced diet provides the necessary nutrients for optimal organ function and disease prevention.

2. Enhanced Mental Health

Physical health and mental health are closely linked, and a healthy lifestyle can have a positive impact on mental health. Exercise releases endorphins, which are known to boost mood and reduce stress, anxiety, and depression. A balanced diet can also help stabilize mood and prevent mental health conditions such as bipolar disorder and schizophrenia.

3. Increased Energy Levels

A healthy lifestyle can also improve energy levels. Regular exercise helps increase stamina and endurance, reducing fatigue and boosting energy levels. A balanced diet provides the necessary nutrients for optimal organ function and cellular metabolism, providing energy for daily activities.

4. Improved Sleep Quality

A healthy lifestyle can improve sleep quality. Exercise helps regulate the circadian rhythm, promoting restful sleep, while a balanced diet provides nutrients that support healthy sleep patterns. A healthy lifestyle also helps reduce stress, anxiety, and depression, which can interfere with sleep quality.

In conclusion, leading a healthy lifestyle has numerous benefits, including improved physical health, enhanced mental health, increased energy levels, and improved sleep quality. A healthy lifestyle requires consistency and effort, but the rewards are worth it. The following chapters of this book will provide a comprehensive guide on how to incorporate exercise and a balanced diet into your daily routine to lead a healthy lifestyle.

Chapter 2:

Good Diet

A good diet is essential for maintaining overall health and well-being. It involves consuming a variety of nutrient-dense foods in the right proportions to support optimal organ function, cellular metabolism, and disease prevention. In this chapter, we will discuss the components of a good diet and how to incorporate them into your daily routine.

Macronutrients

Macronutrients are the three major nutrients that the body needs in large quantities: carbohydrates, protein, and fat. A good diet should contain a balanced ratio of these macronutrients to support optimal organ function and cellular metabolism. Carbohydrates are the primary source of energy for the body, and they should make up approximately 45-65% of daily calorie intake.

Protein is essential for building and repairing tissues, and it should make up approximately 10-35% of daily calorie intake. Fat is important for brain function, hormone production, and insulation, and it should make up approximately 20-35% of daily calorie intake.

Micronutrients

Micronutrients are essential vitamins and minerals that the body needs in small quantities to support optimal organ function and cellular metabolism. A good diet should contain a variety of nutrient-dense foods to ensure adequate intake of micronutrients. Some important micronutrients include vitamin A, vitamin C, vitamin D, calcium, iron, and zinc.

Fiber

Fiber is a type of carbohydrate that the body cannot digest. It is important for maintaining digestive health, regulating blood sugar levels, and reducing the risk of chronic diseases such as heart disease, diabetes, and cancer. A good diet should contain at least 25-30 grams of fiber per day, which can be obtained from fruits, vegetables, whole grains, and legumes.

Water

Water is essential for maintaining proper hydration, regulating body temperature, and flushing toxins from the body. A good diet should include adequate water intake, which varies depending on individual needs and activity level. The general recommendation is to drink at least eight 8-ounce glasses of water per day.

Whole Foods

Whole foods are unprocessed or minimally processed foods that are rich in nutrients and free from additives, preservatives, and artificial ingredients. A good diet should include a variety of whole foods, such as fruits, vegetables, whole grains, lean protein sources, and healthy fats.

In conclusion, a good diet is essential for maintaining overall health and well-being. It should include a balance of macronutrients, micronutrients, fiber, water, and whole foods. The following chapters will provide practical tips on how to incorporate these components into your daily diet to support a healthy lifestyle.

Chapter 3:

Setting Goals

Setting goals is an important step in achieving fitness success. Without clear goals, it can be difficult to stay motivated and focused on your fitness journey. In this chapter, we will discuss the importance of setting goals and provide practical tips on how to set and achieve them.

Why Set Goals?

Setting goals provides a clear direction for your fitness journey. It helps you to identify what you want to achieve and why it is important to you. Goals also help you to track your progress and celebrate your achievements along the way. By setting specific and measurable goals, you can stay motivated and committed to your fitness journey.

How to Set Goals?

When setting fitness goals, it is important to make them specific, measurable, achievable, relevant, and time-bound (SMART). Here are some tips for setting SMART goals:

Be specific: Identify exactly what you want to achieve. For example, instead of setting a goal to "lose weight," set a goal to "lose 10 pounds in the next three months."

Make it measurable: Determine how you will measure progress towards your goal. For example, use a scale to track weight loss progress or a fitness tracker to monitor steps taken or calories burned.

Make it achievable: Set goals that are challenging but realistic. If your goal is too difficult to achieve, it can be demotivating. If it is too easy, you may not feel a sense of accomplishment.

Make it relevant: Ensure that your goals align with your personal values and priorities. If you are not passionate about your goal, it will be difficult to stay motivated.

Make it time-bound: Set a deadline for achieving your goal. This will help you to stay focused and track your progress.

Types of Goals

There are different types of fitness goals that you can set depending on your preferences and needs. Some examples of fitness goals include:

Weight loss: Set a goal to lose a specific amount of weight over a specific period of time.

Strength training: Set a goal to increase the amount of weight you can lift or the number of repetitions you can perform.

Cardiovascular fitness: Set a goal to increase your endurance by running or walking a certain distance or time.

Flexibility: Set a goal to improve your flexibility by performing stretching exercises regularly.

Overall wellness: Set a goal to improve your overall health and well-being by making healthy lifestyle choices.

Strategies for Achieving Goals

Once you have set your fitness goals, it is important to develop a plan to achieve them. Here are some strategies for achieving your fitness goals:

Break it down: Break your goal down into smaller, more manageable steps. This will make it less daunting and easier to achieve.

Make a plan: Develop a plan for achieving your goal, including specific actions you will take and when you will take them.

Track your progress: Keep track of your progress towards your goal. This will help you to stay motivated and make adjustments as needed.

Celebrate your achievements: Celebrate your achievements along the way, no matter how small they may seem. This will help you to stay motivated and committed to your fitness journey.

In conclusion, setting goals is an important step in achieving fitness success. By setting SMART goals, choosing the right types of goals, and developing strategies for achieving them, you can stay motivated and focused on your fitness journey. The following chapters will provide practical tips on how to create a workout plan and make healthy lifestyle choices to support your fitness goals.

Chapter 4:

Creating a Workout Plan

Creating a workout plan is an essential part of getting fit. A well-designed workout plan can help you to achieve your fitness goals, stay motivated, and avoid injury. In this chapter, we will discuss the key components of a workout plan and provide practical tips on how to create one that works for you.

Identify Your Fitness Goals

Before creating a workout plan, it is important to identify your fitness goals. This will help you to tailor your workouts to your specific needs and preferences. For example, if your goal is to improve your cardiovascular fitness, you may want to focus on activities such as running or cycling. If your goal is to build strength, you may want to incorporate weight lifting or resistance training into your workouts.

Choose Your Activities

Once you have identified your fitness goals, it is time to choose the activities that will help you to achieve them. It is important to choose activities that you enjoy and that you are able to do safely. Some popular activities that can be incorporated into a workout plan include:

Cardiovascular exercises: Running, cycling, swimming, and walking.

Strength training: Weight lifting, resistance training, and bodyweight exercises.

Flexibility exercises: Yoga, stretching, and Pilates.

Plan Your Workouts

After choosing your activities, it is time to plan your workouts. A well-designed workout plan should include the following components:

Warm-up: Start with a 5-10 minute warm-up to prepare your body for exercise. This can include light cardio, such as walking or jogging, and dynamic stretching.

Cardiovascular exercise: Aim for at least 30 minutes of cardiovascular exercise per workout, three to five times per week. This can include activities such as running, cycling, or swimming.

Strength training: Incorporate strength training exercises two to three times per week. This can include weight lifting, resistance training, or bodyweight exercises.

Flexibility exercises: Finish your workout with 5-10 minutes of stretching or yoga to improve flexibility and reduce the risk of injury.

Rest days: Allow your body time to rest and recover between workouts. Aim for at least one or two rest days per week.

Make Adjustments

As you progress in your fitness journey, it is important to make adjustments to your workout plan as needed. This may include increasing the intensity or duration of your workouts, adding new exercises or activities, or changing your workout schedule. It is important to listen to your body and make adjustments gradually to avoid injury.

Seek Professional Advice

If you are new to exercise or have specific health concerns, it is important to seek professional advice before starting a workout plan. A certified personal trainer or fitness professional can help you to create a safe and effective workout plan that is tailored to your needs and goals.

In conclusion, creating a workout plan is an essential part of getting fit. By identifying your fitness goals, choosing the right activities, planning your workouts, making adjustments, and seeking professional advice, you can create a workout plan that works for you and helps you to achieve your fitness goals. The next chapter will discuss the importance of nutrition and provide practical tips on how to make healthy food choices to support your fitness journey.

Chapter 5:

Nutrition for Fitness

Nutrition is a crucial component of a healthy lifestyle and can greatly impact your fitness journey. In this chapter, we will discuss the importance of nutrition for fitness and provide practical tips on how to make healthy food choices to support your fitness goals.

Understanding Macronutrients

Macronutrients are the three main nutrients that our body needs in large quantities: carbohydrates, proteins, and fats. Each macronutrient serves a specific purpose in the body, and a balanced diet should include a combination of all three.

Carbohydrates: Carbohydrates are the primary source of energy for the body. They are found in foods such as fruits, vegetables, whole grains, and legumes.

Proteins: Proteins are essential for building and repairing tissues in the body. They are found in foods such as meat, poultry, fish, beans, and nuts.

Fats: Fats are essential for the absorption of certain vitamins and minerals, and for providing energy to the body. They are found in foods such as nuts, seeds, oils, and fatty fish.

Importance of Hydration

Water is essential for maintaining optimal health and fitness. It plays a vital role in regulating body temperature, transporting nutrients, and removing waste products from the body. Aim to drink at least 8-10 cups of water per day, and increase your intake if you are exercising or in hot weather.

Pre- and Post-Workout Nutrition

The timing and composition of your meals can greatly impact your performance during exercise and your recovery afterwards. Aim to eat a small meal or snack that contains a combination of carbohydrates and protein 1-2 hours before exercising to provide your body with energy. After exercising, aim to consume a meal or snack that contains carbohydrates and protein within 30-60 minutes to help replenish energy stores and promote muscle recovery.

Healthy Food Choices

Making healthy food choices can greatly support your fitness journey. Aim to incorporate a variety of fruits, vegetables, whole grains, lean proteins, and healthy fats into your diet. Limit processed foods, sugary drinks, and foods high in saturated fats and sodium.

Portion Control

Portion control is important for maintaining a healthy weight and ensuring that you are consuming the right amount of nutrients. Use measuring cups or a food scale to measure your portions, and be mindful of your serving sizes when eating out.

In conclusion, nutrition is a crucial component of a healthy lifestyle and can greatly impact your fitness journey. By understanding macronutrients, staying hydrated, focusing on pre- and post-workout nutrition, making healthy food choices, and practicing portion control, you can support your fitness goals and maintain optimal health. The next chapter will discuss the importance of lifestyle changes and provide practical tips on how to incorporate healthy habits into your daily routine.

Chapter 6:

Lifestyle Changes for Fitness

Leading a healthy lifestyle is not just about exercise and nutrition, but also about making healthy choices in all aspects of your life. In this chapter, we will discuss the importance of lifestyle changes for fitness and provide practical tips on how to incorporate healthy habits into your daily routine.

Sleep

Sleep plays a crucial role in maintaining optimal health and fitness. Aim to get at least 7-8 hours of sleep per night, and establish a regular sleep routine by going to bed and waking up at the same time every day.

Stress Management

Stress can have negative impacts on both physical and mental health. Practice stress management techniques such as meditation, deep breathing, yoga, or journaling to help manage stress levels and promote relaxation.

Active Lifestyle

Incorporating physical activity into your daily routine can greatly support your fitness goals. Aim to walk or bike instead of driving, take the stairs instead of the elevator, and find ways to be active throughout the day, such as taking regular breaks to stretch or do a quick workout.

Mindful Eating

Mindful eating involves being present and aware while eating, and listening to your body's hunger and fullness cues. Practice mindful eating by eating slowly, without distractions, and paying attention to your body's signals of hunger and fullness.

Social Support

Having a supportive social network can greatly impact your ability to maintain healthy habits. Surround yourself with friends and family who encourage and support your fitness journey, and consider joining a fitness class or finding a workout buddy to keep you motivated.

In conclusion, incorporating healthy lifestyle changes into your daily routine is crucial for maintaining optimal health and fitness. By prioritizing sleep, managing stress, being active, practicing mindful eating, and seeking social support, you can make sustainable lifestyle changes that support your fitness goals. The next chapter will provide tips on how to stay motivated and overcome common barriers to fitness.

Chapter 7:

Staying Motivated and Overcoming Barriers to Fitness

While getting started on a fitness journey can be exciting, staying motivated over time can be a challenge. In this chapter, we will discuss tips on how to stay motivated and overcome common barriers to fitness.

Set Realistic Goals

Setting realistic and achievable goals is important for staying motivated. Break your fitness goals down into smaller, achievable steps and celebrate your progress along the way.

Find an Accountability Partner

Having an accountability partner, such as a friend or family member, can help keep you on track and motivated. Share your goals with them and check in regularly to discuss progress and challenges.

Mix Up Your Routine

Doing the same workout routine day after day can become monotonous and lead to boredom. Mix up your routine by trying new exercises or activities to keep things interesting and challenging.

Track Your Progress

Keeping track of your progress can help you stay motivated and see how far you have come. Consider keeping a fitness journal or using a fitness tracking app to monitor your progress and set new goals.

Overcoming Barriers

Common barriers to fitness include lack of time, motivation, and resources. Overcome these barriers by planning ahead, finding ways to stay motivated, and utilizing resources such as workout videos or fitness classes.

Celebrate Your Achievements

Celebrate your achievements, no matter how small. Acknowledge the hard work and dedication it takes to make healthy lifestyle changes and reward yourself for reaching your goals.

In conclusion, staying motivated and overcoming barriers to fitness is crucial for long-term success. By setting realistic goals, finding an accountability partner, mixing up your routine, tracking your progress, and celebrating your achievements, you can stay motivated and achieve your fitness goals.

Chapter 8:

Advanced Fitness Techniques and Strategies

Once you have established a solid foundation of fitness habits and achieved your initial fitness goals, you may want to explore more advanced techniques and strategies to take your fitness to the next level. In this chapter, we will discuss some advanced fitness techniques and strategies that can help you continue to progress and challenge yourself.

High-Intensity Interval Training (HIIT)

HIIT involves alternating periods of high-intensity exercise with periods of rest or low-intensity exercise. This type of training can be a great way to challenge your body and improve cardiovascular fitness.

Strength Training

Strength training involves using resistance, such as weights or resistance bands, to build and tone muscles. Incorporating strength training into your workout routine can help increase muscle mass, improve bone density, and boost metabolism.

Cross-Training

Cross-training involves incorporating a variety of different types of exercise into your routine, such as running, swimming, and cycling. This can help prevent boredom and overuse injuries while improving overall fitness.

Flexibility and Mobility Training

Flexibility and mobility training involve exercises that improve range of motion and joint mobility. Incorporating stretching and mobility exercises into your routine can help prevent injury and improve overall athletic performance.

Sports-Specific Training

If you participate in a particular sport or activity, sports-specific training can help improve your performance. This type of training involves exercises and drills that mimic the movements and demands of the sport or activity.

Nutrition and Supplementation

As you advance in your fitness journey, paying attention to nutrition and supplementation can become increasingly important. Consulting with a registered dietitian or sports nutritionist can help you develop a nutrition plan that supports your fitness goals. Additionally, supplements such as protein powders, creatine, and pre-workout can provide additional support for muscle growth and performance.

In conclusion, exploring advanced fitness techniques and strategies can help you continue to progress and challenge yourself. Incorporating HIIT, strength training, cross-training, flexibility and mobility training, sports-specific training, and paying attention to nutrition and supplementation can help you achieve your fitness goals and maintain a healthy and active lifestyle.

Chapter 9:

Overcoming Fitness Plateaus

At some point in your fitness journey, you may experience a plateau where you no longer see progress despite your best efforts. This can be frustrating and discouraging, but there are strategies you can use to overcome fitness plateaus and continue making progress towards your goals.

Reassess Your Goals

It's important to regularly reassess your goals and make sure they are still relevant and achievable. If you've been working towards the same goal for a long time, it may be time to set new goals and challenge yourself in new ways.

Mix Up Your Routine

If you've been doing the same workouts and exercises for a long time, your body may have adapted and become too efficient at them. Mixing up your routine can challenge your body in new ways and help break through a plateau. Try new exercises, change the order of your workouts, or try a different type of exercise altogether.

Increase Intensity or Volume

If you've been doing the same workouts for a long time, you may need to increase the intensity or volume to continue making progress. This can be done by increasing the weight or resistance, increasing the number of sets or repetitions, or reducing rest time between sets.

Get Rest and Recovery

Overtraining can lead to fatigue and injury, which can stall progress. Make sure to prioritize rest and recovery by taking rest days, getting enough sleep, and practicing self-care techniques like stretching, foam rolling, and massage.

Nutrition and Hydration

Proper nutrition and hydration are essential for making progress in fitness. Make sure you are fueling your body with enough calories and nutrients to support your workouts, and staying hydrated throughout the day.

In conclusion, fitness plateaus can be frustrating, but they are a natural part of the fitness journey. By reassessing your goals, mixing up your routine, increasing intensity or volume, prioritizing rest and recovery, and paying attention to nutrition and hydration, you can overcome plateaus and continue making progress towards your goals.

Chapter 10:

Maintaining Your Fitness Level

Congratulations! You've worked hard and achieved your fitness goals. But the journey doesn't end there. Maintaining your fitness level is just as important as achieving it. Here are some tips for maintaining your fitness level:

Set New Goals

Setting new goals can help keep you motivated and focused. Whether it's running a faster 5K, lifting heavier weights, or trying a new fitness activity, having something to work towards can keep you on track.

Continue with Regular Exercise

Don't stop exercising just because you've achieved your goals. Regular exercise is essential for maintaining your fitness level. Try to exercise at least 3-4 times a week and include a variety of activities to keep it interesting.

Adjust Your Routine

As you get stronger and fitter, you may need to adjust your routine to continue making progress. This can include increasing the weight or resistance, changing up your exercises, or adding in new types of workouts.

Monitor Your Progress

Keep track of your progress and monitor your fitness level regularly. This can help you identify any areas where you may need to make changes to your routine.

Prioritize Rest and Recovery

Just like during your fitness journey, rest and recovery are essential for maintaining your fitness level. Make sure to prioritize rest days, get enough sleep, and practice self-care techniques to prevent injury and burnout.

Healthy Nutrition

Maintaining a healthy diet is just as important as exercise in maintaining your fitness level. Make sure you are fueling your body with enough nutrients to support your workouts, and avoid l

In conclusion, maintaining your fitness level is an ongoing process that requires commitment and effort. By setting new goals, continuing with regular exercise, adjusting your routine, monitoring your progress, prioritizing rest and recovery, and maintaining a healthy diet, you can maintain your fitness level and enjoy the many benefits of a healthy lifestyle.

Chapter 11:

Overcoming Common Fitness Obstacles

Even the most dedicated fitness enthusiasts face obstacles from time to time that can derail their progress. Here are some common obstacles and how to overcome them:

Lack of Motivation

Sometimes, it can be hard to stay motivated to exercise regularly. To overcome this obstacle, try setting small, achievable goals and rewarding yourself when you reach them. Also, consider finding a workout buddy or joining a fitness class to help keep you accountable.

Time Constraints

Busy schedules can make it difficult to find time to exercise. To overcome this obstacle, try incorporating exercise into your daily routine. For example, take the stairs instead of the elevator, walk or bike to work, or do a quick workout during your lunch break.

Injury

Injuries can be frustrating and discouraging, but it's important to listen to your body and allow yourself time to heal. To overcome this obstacle, seek medical advice and follow a rehabilitation plan. You may need to modify your workout routine temporarily or try low-impact exercises until you fully recover.

Plateaus

Hitting a plateau in your fitness progress can be discouraging, but it's normal. To overcome this obstacle, try changing up your routine or adding in new types of workouts to challenge your body. Also, make sure you are getting enough rest and nutrition to support your workouts.

Lack of Confidence

Lack of confidence can make it difficult to try new workouts or go to the gym. To overcome this obstacle, start with small steps, such as trying a new workout at home or going to the gym during less crowded times. Remember, everyone starts somewhere and it's okay to make mistakes or ask for help.

In conclusion, common fitness obstacles can be overcome with the right mindset and strategies. By setting small, achievable goals, incorporating exercise into your daily routine, seeking medical advice for injuries, changing up your routine to avoid plateaus, and building confidence through small steps, you can overcome obstacles and achieve your fitness goals.

Chapter 12:

Staying Motivated for Long-Term Success

Maintaining long-term fitness success requires ongoing motivation and commitment. Here are some tips to help you stay motivated:

Set Realistic Goals

Setting realistic goals that are achievable within a specific timeframe can help keep you motivated. Break down larger goals into smaller, manageable ones and celebrate each milestone along the way.

Track Your Progress

Tracking your progress can help you see how far you've come and keep you motivated to keep going. Use a fitness tracker or journal to record your workouts and progress over time.

Find an Accountability Partner

Having someone to hold you accountable and encourage you can make a big difference in staying motivated. Find a workout buddy or hire a personal trainer to help keep you on track.

Mix Up Your Routine

Doing the same workout every day can get boring and lead to a lack of motivation. Mix up your routine by trying new workouts or changing the intensity or duration of your current ones.

Reward Yourself

Rewarding yourself for reaching milestones or sticking to your fitness routine can help keep you motivated. Treat yourself to a massage, new workout clothes, or a healthy meal at your favorite restaurant.

Focus on the Benefits

Reminding yourself of the benefits of exercise, such as increased energy, improved mood, and better overall health, can help keep you motivated on days when you don't feel like working out.

Stay Positive

Positive self-talk and mindset can make a big difference in staying motivated. Focus on the progress you've made and the goals you've achieved rather than dwelling on setbacks or obstacles.

In conclusion, staying motivated for long-term fitness success requires commitment and ongoing effort. By setting realistic goals, tracking progress, finding an accountability partner, mixing up your routine, rewarding yourself, focusing on the benefits, and staying positive, you can stay motivated and achieve your fitness goals.

Chapter 13:

Overcoming Plateaus and Setbacks

It's not uncommon to hit a plateau or experience setbacks on your fitness journey. Here are some tips to help you overcome them:

Change Your Routine

If you've hit a plateau in your progress, changing up your workout routine can help. Try incorporating new exercises or changing the intensity, duration, or frequency of your workouts.

Reassess Your Goals

If you're experiencing setbacks, it may be helpful to reassess your goals and adjust them if necessary.

Maybe you need to set more realistic goals, or maybe you need to challenge yourself more.

Take a Break

Sometimes taking a break from your routine can be helpful. This can give your body time to rest and recover, and can also help you come back to your routine with renewed energy and motivation.

Focus on Nutrition

Nutrition plays a big role in fitness success, so if you're experiencing setbacks, take a look at your diet. Are you getting enough of the right nutrients? Are you eating too many unhealthy foods? Making changes to your diet can help you break through a plateau or overcome setbacks.

Get Support

If you're struggling with setbacks or plateaus, it can be helpful to get support from others. Join a fitness group or hire a personal trainer to help you stay on track and overcome obstacles.

Stay Positive

It's important to stay positive and not get discouraged by setbacks or plateaus. Remind yourself of the progress you've made so far and focus on the positive changes you're making for your health and well-being.

In conclusion, hitting a plateau or experiencing setbacks is a common part of the fitness journey. By changing your routine, reassessing your goals, taking a break, focusing on nutrition, getting support, and staying positive, you can overcome these obstacles and continue to make progress towards your fitness goals.

Chapter 14:

Maintaining Your Fitness Journey

Now that you've achieved your fitness goals, the next step is to maintain your progress and make fitness a lifelong habit. Here are some tips to help you maintain your fitness journey:

Set New Goals

Setting new fitness goals can help you maintain your progress and continue to challenge yourself. Whether it's running a 5K or learning a new exercise, setting new goals can help you stay motivated and engaged.

Mix Up Your Workouts

Keeping your workouts varied and interesting can help you maintain your fitness routine. Try new exercises, take different classes, or switch up your workout location to keep things fresh.

Stay Consistent

Staying consistent with your workouts is key to maintaining your progress. Try to stick to a regular schedule and make exercise a non-negotiable part of your daily routine.

Prioritize Recovery

Recovery is just as important as exercise when it comes to maintaining your fitness journey. Make sure to incorporate rest days, stretch regularly, and prioritize sleep to give your body the time it needs to recover and repair.

Celebrate Your Successes

Don't forget to celebrate your successes and acknowledge how far you've come on your fitness journey. Take pride in your progress and use it as motivation to continue on your path towards a healthy and active lifestyle.

Find a Support System

Having a support system can help you stay motivated and accountable. Whether it's a workout buddy, a coach, or a fitness community, finding people who share your passion for fitness can help you stay on track.

In conclusion, maintaining your fitness journey requires dedication, consistency, and a willingness to continue challenging yourself. By setting new goals, mixing up your workouts, staying consistent, prioritizing recovery, celebrating your successes, and finding a support system, you can make fitness a lifelong habit and continue to reap the benefits of a healthy and active lifestyle.

Chapter 15:

Overcoming Common Fitness Challenges

Despite your best efforts, you may encounter common fitness challenges along your journey. Here are some tips to help you overcome them:

Lack of Motivation

It's normal to experience a lack of motivation from time to time. To overcome this challenge, try setting smaller, achievable goals, finding a workout buddy, or treating yourself to a new workout outfit or equipment.

Plateauing Progress

If you feel like you've hit a plateau in your progress, it may be time to mix up your workout routine, increase the intensity or duration of your workouts, or try a new form of exercise.

Time Constraints

Balancing work, family, and social commitments can make it difficult to find time for exercise. To overcome this challenge, try scheduling your workouts ahead of time, finding a gym or workout facility close to your workplace or home, or breaking your workouts into smaller, more manageable sessions throughout the day.

Injuries

Injuries can be frustrating and can set back your progress. To overcome this challenge, focus on injury prevention by warming up properly, using proper form during exercises, and incorporating low-impact exercises into your routine. If you do experience an injury, seek medical attention and modify your workouts as necessary.

Lack of Knowledge or Resources

If you feel like you lack the knowledge or resources to achieve your fitness goals, consider hiring a personal trainer, taking a fitness class, or utilizing online resources to learn more about exercise and nutrition.

Remember, every fitness journey is unique and comes with its own set of challenges. By staying focused on your goals, seeking support when needed, and being flexible in your approach, you can overcome common fitness challenges and continue to make progress towards a healthier, more active lifestyle.

Chapter 18:

Maintaining Your Progress

Congratulations on reaching your fitness goals! However, maintaining your progress can be just as challenging as achieving it. Here are some tips for staying on track and continuing to lead a healthy lifestyle:

Set New Goals

Once you've achieved your initial goals, it's important to set new ones to keep yourself motivated and focused. These goals can be anything from running a 5K to lifting a certain amount of weight.

Keep a Workout Schedule

Maintain a regular workout schedule to ensure that you stay consistent with your exercise routine. Consider working with a trainer or finding a workout buddy to help you stay accountable.

Track Your Progress

Continue to track your progress, whether it's through measurements, photos, or fitness apps. This can help you see how far you've come and identify areas for improvement.

Make Healthy Choices

Continue to make healthy choices when it comes to your diet and lifestyle. Focus on whole, nutrient-dense foods and limit processed and sugary foods. Additionally, aim to get enough sleep and manage your stress levels.

Stay Flexible

Remember to stay flexible and adaptable in your fitness journey. Life can throw curveballs, so it's important to be able to adjust your workouts and goals accordingly.

By following these tips and maintaining a consistent and healthy lifestyle, you can continue to make progress and reach new levels of fitness and wellness.

Chapter 19:

Common Fitness Mistakes to Avoid

When it comes to getting fit, there are some common mistakes that many people make. Here are a few to watch out for:

Overtraining

While consistency is important, it's equally important to give your body time to rest and recover. Overtraining can lead to injury and burnout.

Focusing Too Much on Cardio

While cardio is important for cardiovascular health, strength training is also crucial for building muscle and boosting your metabolism.

Not Eating Enough

Restricting calories too much can actually slow down your metabolism and make it harder to lose weight. Make sure you're fueling your body with enough calories to support your workouts and daily activities.

Relying Too Much on Supplements

Supplements can be helpful, but they're not a magic solution. Make sure you're getting your nutrients from whole, nutrient-dense foods and not relying solely on supplements.

Comparing Yourself to Others

Everyone's fitness journey is different, so avoid comparing yourself to others. Focus on your own progress and celebrate your achievements.

By avoiding these common fitness mistakes and focusing on a balanced, sustainable approach to fitness, you can set yourself up for success and reach your goals.

Chapter 20:

Conclusion

Congratulations! You've made it to the end of this book on how to get fit. By now, you should have a good understanding of the importance of leading a healthy lifestyle, the benefits of exercise and a balanced diet, and how to create a workout plan that works for you.

Remember, getting fit is a journey, not a destination. It takes time, dedication, and hard work. But the rewards are worth it – improved health, increased energy, and a better quality of life.

In conclusion, we hope this book has provided you with the knowledge and tools to take control of your health and fitness, and to achieve your fitness goals. Whether you're just starting out or looking to take your fitness to the next level, remember to be patient, consistent, and enjoy the journey.

Thank you for reading, and we wish you all the best on your fitness journey!

9 798390 347829